A Doula's Guide to Menstruation

By Jemmais Keval-Baxter
The Ho'oponopono Doula™

Published by Matrilineal Ink

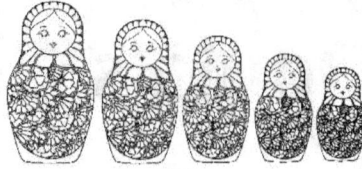

Matrilineal Ink

www.matrilineal.cl

Published by: Matrilineal Ink™
www.matrilineal.cl
ISBN: 978-1-9998071-6-0

A Doula's Guide to Menstruation

By Jemmais Keval-Baxter
The Ho'oponopono Doula™

Published by Matrilineal Ink

Matrilineal Ink

www.matrilineal.cl

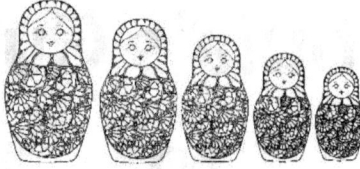

Other books in the series include:

A Doula's Guide to Nutrition
A Doula's Guide to The Placenta
A Doula's Guide to Breastfeeding
A Doula's Guide to Education

Also, by Jemmais Keval-Baxter Ho'oponopono Birth: Meditations on Ho'oponopono for Pregnancy and Childbirth

Table of Contents

Introduction

The average woman will bleed once a month for 25+ years. Menstruation is a part of our daily lives, and it is part of a cycle that unites all women, linking us with our ancestors. It affects the relationships that we have with ourselves, our parents, our children, our siblings, our peers, our jobs, our partners our lives, and our society as a whole.

Regardless of the significant role menstruation plays in our lives, it is such a taboo, such a hushed and controversial subject that even advertisements for menstrual hygiene products are obscured in mystery and euphemisms. The most we are likely to hear about menstruation as we are growing up is negative propaganda, regarding menstrual cramps, mood swings and comfort craving that end in chocolate binges, Menstruation is a joke or worse it is a curse.

Underneath the ignorance and bigotry left over from thousands of years of religiously dogmatic patriarchal paradigms, modern women are beginning to rediscover the ancient blood mysteries that moved their bodies in time with the cosmos, the oceans, creativity, and life on earth. When we understand our menstruation, we know our fertility, and we understand a very vital part of ourselves and who we are in relation to this world, our bodies, and our identities. As women, our gender identity is intimately linked to our biological imperative to reproduce, we are creative, nurturing sources of life and healing. Let us discover the secrets of menstruation that have been hidden away from us for so long so that we can reawaken our blood wisdom and share it with generations to come.

Menstrual Cycle and Seasons

A woman's menstrual cycle is intimately linked to her fertility and to the relationship that she has with herself, her body and her identity as a woman.

Menstruation is seen as a taboo in modern culture, and in many other patriarchal societies, the great potential of the womb to provide wisdom, healing, and harmony with the cycles and seasons of the natural world have been oppressed and forgotten for millennia. Today we are sold sanitary products that effectively allow women to carry on with their lives as if they were not experiencing menstruation at all. This is often cited as a benefit, yet it benefits the rhythm and structure of an industrial society that values interchangeable productive employees, rather than honoring and helping the natural rhythm of the woman herself.

Women have been menstruating since the beginning of time. We are womb-men because we have a womb, and the language of the womb is our ancient tongue. Though many have tried to ignore and suppress its voice and its influence, it can never be eradicated, for the womb is the seat of all fertility and creativity, without it, our species would cease to exist.

There was a time that the rhythm of the womb was respected and honored by every member of society. Early cultures were founded upon these rhythms that linked us to the cosmos, and the 28-day monthly cycle that connected every woman to the celestial heavens and the influence of the moon unified us as a sex and set us in harmony with our environment.

It was this easily identifiable and quantifiable cycle that founded our understanding and measurement of time, astronomy and geometry, forming the basis of the first calendars; 13 moons, or menstrual cycles per year, 4x 7day phases to each cycle (and laying the foundations for the week). Even the 266 days of fetal gestation greatly influenced the Mayan calendar.

So much of our early understanding of ourselves and the universe came from observations of nature. However, in our arrogance and ignorance, centuries later we oppress, suppress and overlook our natural rhythms and the harmonious influence of nature, and in doing so, we have lost a great deal of wisdom, known to our ancestors, and knowledge of how to live sustainably and contentedly within our world. We have also created a disharmony within our own bodies, which has negatively affected the health and well-being of thousands of women around the globe.

How could we ever assume that a pattern so profound and constant in our expression of life in the universe could be inconsequential?

Women no longer have the support and experience of their elders to teach them the deep and profound secrets of menstruation. So much of ancient feminine wisdom has been intentionally destroyed through the dominating influence of patriarchal and imperial colonization; we can only hope to recover and rediscover a small portion of the knowledge lost to us. By observing ourselves, and by consulting the collective wisdom of the female sisterhood, we may yet hear that voice which comes from the depth of our womb and speaks to us with ageless, limitless insight, providing truths we have long forgotten.

Women make up half of the world. Something which affects half of the population is hugely significant and deserves to be understood and applied in our daily lives. Our daughters must identify with themselves, and their place in the cycle of the universe. Their passage through puberty into adolescence and the initiation of menarche should be celebrated and honored, as it still is in many indigenous societies. Sons and fathers need to be educated to understand the rhythms of the mysterious female creatures that inhabit their world, their lives, and their families. Males should be taught to respect their sisters, mothers, wives, and daughters, thus, learning the actual value of women and the honor they deserve.

Unless men and women are educated as to what it entails to be womb-man, as well as what it genuinely means to be a man, then we can never hope to honor ourselves and cultivate a harmonious society together.

People come in two varieties, male and female, for a reason. There is a harmony in this duality, no man is the same as a woman, and no woman is the same as a man, it would be pointless if we were interchangeable, and only suppresses and denies our valuable gifts. We each have something vital to contribute.

Admittedly, it would be more efficient to have one sex that was capable of self-replication, and yet this is not what we have, nor what we were given. Only in honoring and valuing all the aspects of our beings can we embrace them and make use of their positive application in a society that functions to the credit and benefit of all.

28 Days

The menstrual cycle follows a roughly 28-day cycle, which can be further refined into four distinct phases, or seasons, each lasting an average of seven days. Every woman will experience a different length of her menstrual cycle, and the timing of the passage that she takes through these phases will be blurred.

It is necessary for every woman to observe and understand her own cycle to incorporate the benefit revealed by following the menstrual phases. The phases identified in this book are just guidelines that may need to be adapted to the individual.

The menstrual cycle is greatly influenced by the lunar cycle and our rhythmic exposure to light at night. During the new moon, nights are very dark. The moon slowly waxes over a 14-day period culminating in the full moon, which provides the most considerable amount of night-time illumination. From this abundant pregnancy, the moon then wanes, providing less light each night until the dark of the moon, and the new moon returns.

Women's ovulation is timed with the full moon. However, modern light and conveniences such as electricity and artificial lighting, especially in cities, can overwhelm our systems, and put our body clocks out of balance. Many women find that their menstrual cycles are not synchronized to the sequence of the moon, and this can negatively affect fertility. Conversely, women who live in the countryside, spend a lot of time in nature, or make a conscious effort to pay attention to the moon cycle, often find that their menstrual cycle adjusts itself to this default pattern very quickly.

The medical industry measures the menstrual cycle from the first day of bleeding, labeling this as day one of the menstrual cycle. Women bleed for different amounts of time, often correlated to weight and diet, with more substantial flows reported by carnivores than vegans and more extended or heavier periods reported by women that carry more adipose tissue.

Malnourishment and inadequate fat stores in the body will force the body to recognize that it is incapable of supporting new life, and so periods often cease. This phenomenon is known to many anorexics and people with eating disorders as well as practitioners of yoga that follow stringent minimalistic diets and professional athletes that consume all of the energy that they can feed into their body, very quickly.

Day one may not be during the same phase of the moon for everyone. However, the first day after bleeding is likely to correspond to the date of the new moon.

Menstruation (days 1-7) - Winter –

Dark/New Moon - Crone

Pre-Ovulation (days 7-14) - Spring –

Waxing Moon - Maiden

Ovulation (days 14-21) - Summer - Full

Moon - Mother

Pre-Menstruation (days 21-28) - Autumn –

Waning Moon – Maga

Ovulation is considered to occur 14 days before the first day of bleeding, however, some women with irregular periods have shorter lengths between ovulation and cleansing; this greatly decreases their fertility as it does not provide the optimal opportunity for a fertilized egg to implant into the uterus.

Restoring balance to the menstrual cycle is very important and will increase reproductive balance which can promote fertility and also relieve health issues relating to hormone imbalances such as acne, menstrual cramps, and mood swings. Adequate nutrition, rest, relaxation (stress can be very detrimental), and specific herbal remedies can be very effective at restoring equilibrium. Milk Vetch Root, Chinese angelica root, vitex (chaste berry), Chinese foxglove root, and Gogi berries are highly recommended by Ni, Daoshing, Herko, Dana in his book The Tao of Fertility. Red Clover and Red Raspberry (leaf and fruit) are well-known herbs available through western herbal medicine and confirmed by Susan Weed in Wise Woman Herbal for the Childbearing Years. While you can easily increase the number of raspberries, goji berries or other berries (they are powerhouses of vitamins, minerals, antioxidants, and other vital nutrients), I recommend consulting a professional herbal medicine or Chinese herbal medicine practitioner, who can recommend a course of treatment that is specifically adapted to your needs as an individual.

Spring, Day 7-14 (Maiden)

After the bleeding, cleansing time of menstruation, the energy of woman awakens, like the warming of the earth at the beginning of spring, after the cold dormant restful period of winter. Many women experience an increase in energy at this time, as well as feeling physically lighter. They also feel jubilant, inspired and dynamic, ready to start new projects and implement positive changes and healthy habits in their lives. This phase has been likened to the energy of the young girl, the prepubescent, the virgin who has boundless enthusiasm, motivation, and drive. Many women feel that this is a time of peak physical performance for sports and athleticism.

Summer, Day 14-21 (Mother)

Ovulation and incubation. This phase is a time of nurturing, or creativity and manifestation. Our thoughts and energies are focused outwards, and we are naturally inclined to be generous to others with our time and resources. We are more inclined to be sociable and are naturally designed to radiate beauty and attract attention from the opposite sex. As intimate relations are more likely to resort in pregnancy at this time, women may also experience an increase in libido. All our hormones are saying yes, so it is essential to be cautious at this time and not let ourselves get carried away unless we mean it.

This is also a time of increased patience, dedication, and caring for the needs of those around us. This a great time to explore arts and crafts and to share creativity with your community and family through sewing projects as well as every type of collaborative and group work. We are experiencing the phase of the mother, and also the wife, so it is natural for us to use our time to create projects with our children, enjoy spending time with them, helping them with their homework or work together in the garden. Interpersonal relationships of all kinds will benefit from your understanding and attention at this time.

Autumn, Day 21-28 (Maga)

Pre-menstrual. Unless your body has achieved its goal of becoming pregnant, then the autumn phase of the cycle will be expressed through a withdrawing of energy from the outer world, and more focus will be on personal reflection, self-care, and reevaluation. This is often the phase least understood by women and society, (and most feared by Patriarchal institutions, as demonstrated through the vilification of witches and sorceresses during the witch-burning that continues in our time throughout the world).

It is a time of selfishness, as opposed to the selfless giving of attention and energy and effort of the spring and summer phases, this is the occasion to dedicate to one's self. It is also a time of disappointment. Our biological efforts for fertility have been unsuccessful, and our thoughts and evaluations can seem critical, frustrations may rise to the surface, and our energies can easily be misinterpreted as destructive.

This phase, however, is not negative. It is natural for us to experience these energies, they serve a beneficial purpose. We are no longer so concerned with the thoughts and feelings of others that we bite our tongue for the sake of maintaining peace. Instead, we unleash the full force of our frank and unflattering appraisals, we attack our self-image and apply our scrutiny to others and the world around us. We scrap projects that we feel are unsuccessful; we clean our house, we nag our partners and rebel against the limitations and expectations of social and religious structure and tackle every area of our lives with ruthless cleansing. The reason that we do this is because we are seeking to remove from our lives anything that is not positive, constructive or productive. We are cleansing our lives of all the rubbish (including insincerity) as we banish unhealthy people, thought patterns, habits and relationships from our lives with brutal honesty.

Understanding this phase, and the underlying positive intentions of this energy can be very helpful in keeping our reactions within safe and constructive boundaries. Acknowledging our feelings, but also recognizing the capacity for their exaggeration at this time can help prevent us from getting carried away and doing or saying something we may later regret. Sometimes it is easier to avoid people and situations that we simply do not have the patience or diplomacy to deal with during this time and restrict our social activities and obligations. It is also important not to be too hard on ourselves. If there is something about ourselves that we feel is not working, then it is possible to take this opportunity as positive motivation for a change. Begin cleansing the cigarettes/ junk food/ mess/ abusive relationships/ unhealthy working conditions (or whatever) from our lives during this phase, in order to start afresh with the energy and enthusiasm of the next spring phase.

Winter, Day 21-28 (Crone)

Menstruation. This is a phase of dormancy, rest, cleansing, wisdom, perspective, and reflection. Women have been gifted with a unique opportunity to detox their bodies once a month through menstruation. Many cultures and religions to this day, continue to impose restrictions and taboos upon women during their menstruation, which were initially developed to honor the needs of our bodies at this time.

Withdrawal from the community during menstruation, into what is often referred to as a moon lodge, provided women with an opportunity to rest from the usual routine of cooking, cleaning, and attending to the needs of their family and household. It also restricted sexual relations (often a welcome relief in cultures where marital relations are considered a husband's right and a woman's obligation, rather than a gift and privilege for which the woman has the right to choose to share or decline at will).

Restriction of the diet to fruits and vegetables often aided in the body's cleansing process and provided an obligatory opportunity for every woman's body to rest and heal. The meditative focus of women at this time was also cultivated as an opportunity to communicate with the divine, where women provided the opportunity to listen without other distractions or obligations, were able to receive visions, prophetic dreams, insights and epiphanies. Native American cultures often awaited the collective wisdom of the women emerging from the moon lodges, where dreams and visions were compared, analyzed and shared with the community. Providing advice on how to improve daily life for the community, from where and when to move camp, what animals to hunt (and what animals to leave to restore their numbers), new inventions, healing medicines, and many other contributions. During this phase, every woman could connect with their inner crone and be consulted with the respect typically awarded to the elder women who had passed through menstruation and into menopause.

Crones

"The Great Mother was the earth, as well as the sea, the moon, the Milky Way, the elements, mountains, rivers, animistic or non-representational, stones, vegetation, women, time, fate, intelligence, birth love, and death. Her scriptures credited her with the initial creation of the universe and everything in it, as well as the ongoing creation and temporary preservation of each creature. She was also the destroyer of the universe itself at doomsday, only to prepare a new creation in her next cycle." The Crone, women of age wisdom and power by Barbara G. Walker

Modern society, as a result of thousands of years of intentional persecution of women, and in particular elder, independent women, who no longer served sexual and reproductive purposes, blatantly disregards the post-menopausal woman. Thus, awarding cult status to youth and beauty, and effectively dismissing the old women, who would have been the elders of our communities, delegating them to convalescent homes (along with their male counterparts) where their interaction and influence upon society can be kept to a minimum until they die.

In traditional cultures, elder women/crones were awarded greater status. This recognition was based on their years of experience, acquired knowledge and the benefit of the wisdom that they had achieved by successfully experiencing and surviving all of the previous phases of womanhood and from their insights based on the long observation of people and communities. Elder women often formed advisory councils which dictated and upheld the moral standards and laws of the community. The all-seeing eye of the grandmother, was the omnipresent observer that kept little children in line, even as they grew into adults, and great respect was given to the highest expression of the female which represented Mother Nature our life giver and creative force on Earth.

The elder women's council was often the ultimate authority, confirming or denying the decisions of war councils and other leaders of their communities. No one could dismiss the cumulative wisdom of the collective mother, who cared and watched over her children, throughout the entire length of her life. A mother's love never ends, and the love these women had for their children, people and communities, enabled and motivated them to provide the best possible advice for their descendants to follow and thrive. Our mother's love always wants the best for us.

Many of the prophetesses and oracles of ancient Greece as well as the priestesses in ancient Egypt and other ancient societies, were consulted regarding the visions that they received during their menstruation. Sadly, the visions, insights, and intuition received by women at this time had no place within the dominant patriarchal religions that came afterward, and the gifts associated with being in one's moon house were later denigrated to lunacy and labeled mental health disorders, witchcraft and the work of the devil.

Modern society is not organized to acknowledge the needs of this phase of the menstrual cycle and many women who work and have family obligations find it difficult to withdraw from the world at this time and take the rest that they genuinely need and deserve.

Jane Hardwicke Collings suggests in her article; "The spiritual practice of menstruation" that women would be able to smoothly transition through the autumn phase if they knew that their patience and efforts would be rewarded with a well-earned rest during their menstruation.

Even if you do find it impossible to implement complete withdraw from the world during your menstruation, there are a number of practices that you may consider applying for your self-care. First don't over-schedule yourself, only take on the primary obligations during this time, try to provide uninterrupted time and space for quiet reflection and meditation. If your schedule allows it, this may be an opportunity to explore personal creative projects such as art or writing, where personal insights can be expressed and incorporated into your work.

Treat your body to a healthy detoxifying diet, avoiding all stimulants such as coffee, tea, alcohol, processed food, sugar, nicotine and other toxins. Removing these unhealthy items from the diet has been known to be effective in relieving discomfort and pain for many women experiencing PMS. Try to avoid consuming meat and dairy products at this time, as they can be taxing on the digestive system, and enjoy lots of fresh fruits, vegetables, nuts and seeds and stay hydrated with herbal teas and raw fruit juices.

If you do suffer from discomfort, please try to resist taking pharmaceuticals to mask the pain, as this rarely encourages you to find and address the source of the issue. Instead, try adopting a clean diet, using heat (hot water bottles) rest and alternative medicines such as herbal treatments, acupuncture, and massage, vaginal steams and gentle exercise such as womb yoga or Chi Qung to help restore balance to your reproductive system, and relieve any discomfort. Please seek out a holistic gynecologist, and in the meantime try experimenting with a dairy-free diet, increasing your consumption of zinc and magnesium which have been noted to provide relief and assistance for many women suffering from Endometriosis and Polycystic Ovarian Syndrome, etc.

The reason that many women are advised to refrain from sexual relations during the time of menstruation is because the energy of the womb is in general receptive mode, it receives not just sperm, but much of the energy of the sexual partner. During menstruation the womb is emptying itself, cleansing itself, and like a vacuum or a void has an increased capacity to attract energy at this time, which is not necessarily healthy for the womb. Many women were restricted from participating in ceremonies during menstruation, in native cultures and within the Muslim and Hindu religions amongst others for this very reason. The womb attracted all of the energy being raised during the ceremony, potentially nullifying the tradition and making the menstruating woman vulnerable to illness or possession.

This motivation, was, however, forgotten by many who later misinterpreted the exclusion of menstruating women as a sign of them being unclean or contaminated. Many cultures also warned women not to swim or wash in the river, but rather save any wash water for ceremonial disposal, as the blood was thought to attract and feed predators of the terrestrial and supernatural worlds.

Menstrual blood is extremely powerful energetically. It has always been used ceremonially as an offering to the Mother Earth, whom it fertilizes and nourishes exquisitely and is the original blood given. Blood without sacrifice, since women bleed without wounds or illness, our offering is a blessing to ourselves as much as to the earth as it cleans our bodies and fertilizes the land.

Menstrual Diary

With the above ideas in mind, I recommend observing your menstrual cycle for a minimum of three cycles and keeping a journal. You should take note of the day of menstruation, the phase of the moon, your subjective evaluations of mood, energy levels, thoughts, feelings, health, dreams, cravings, etc. After three cycles, it is very likely that you will begin to see a pattern emerging that reflects your own expression of the various phases of the menstrual cycle. With this information, you will be better prepared to predict and understand the emotional, physical, psychological, sexual and spiritual characteristics and tendencies that you experience during each phase.

Once you are familiar with your individual pattern, then you may find it worthwhile sharing your experiences and observations with friends and family and even seek out a local group of women who explore and honor the menstrual cycle with moon lodges or gatherings where you can share your experiences and advice. Many women feel that after connecting and understanding their personal menstrual cycle and listening to and honoring the needs of each phase, physically, spiritually, mentally and emotionally, that they experience a greater harmony with themselves.

Honoring our bodies and listening to their communications, providing rest and adequate nutrition, goes a long way to addressing their needs; relieving any painful and uncomfortable symptoms associated with menstruation and PMT, which are your body's way of communicating (loudly) its needs to you.

"There are also studies which support the idea that the attitude of furtiveness and shame which surrounds menstruation in our culture is at least partly responsible for the physical discomfort that many women go through each month." In the Blood: the myths, magic, and mystery of moonflow by Spiraldancer.

Acknowledging the honor of your menstruation and understanding its place of wisdom and influence in your life, may contribute to helping you interact positively with this vital part of your womb-self.

The menstrual/fertility cycle of women is so intimately linked to the influence of the moon, that once you become familiar with the lunar rhythm, you may experience the cycling of emotions and attributes associated with each phase of the moon even during pregnancy when your menstrual bleeding is likely to have stopped.

Contraception
The Pill

The majority of women in western society have been persuaded to consider the benefits of the contraceptive pill since its release in the early 1960's. Unfortunately, for a large number of women, from early adolescence until they make the conscious decision to try for a baby, the consumption of the contraceptive pill has meant that they never truly experience natural menstruation. The advantages of the contraceptive pill have been widely publicized and are well known for allowing women to have sexual intercourse whenever they chose, lower risk of pregnancy, and potentially improving one's complexion and relieving some of the symptoms of PMS, even increasing breast size. The disadvantages and side effects, however, are less well known.

The contraceptive pill is an artificial combination of estrogen and progesterone that prevents ovulation, the bleeding which occurs during this artificial cycle is not true menstruation "a pill bleed is a withdrawal bleed dictated by the dosing regimen of the drug manufacturer" Dr. Lara Briden, ND.

Use of the contraceptive pill has been linked to an increased occurrence of cancer, especially breast cancer (that has significantly been on the rise since the introduction of the pill to mainstream "health care"). In addition, there are links to cervical, liver cancer, high blood pressure, blood clots and thrombosis (which are responsible for heart attacks, strokes, and pulmonary embolisms), and lower bone-density resulting in osteoporosis later in life. Although osteoporosis is thought to be an inevitable disadvantage of menopause, its rate of occurrence increases exponentially for menopausal women who took the pill during their fertile years.

Unlike other women who relied on barrier methods of contraception such as the condom, there is a significant increase in the rates of transmission of venereal diseases, including a two-fold increased risk of catching and passing on HIV, and Herpes when using the pill.

The pill is also thought to influence the kind of partner that we are attracted to. Many factors affect our choice of partner; however, from a purely biological perspective, our bodies are programmed to choose partners who are genetically different from ourselves, thus ensuring healthy offspring. Since the brain and the body communicate via hormones, the consumption of artificial hormones (such as those found in the pill) overrides our bodies natural selection, which results in us unable to hear what our body is communicating to us. Studies have linked the effects of the pill to women choosing partners that have genetic material very similar to themselves, which they suggest has led to increased rates of infertility as well as higher rates of unsuccessful long-term relationships.

Young girls (between the ages of 12-15) are now being targeted for birth control almost as soon as they reach menarche (their first period), "Menarche is also when girls start to make female hormones for the first time." Says Dr. Lara Briden, ND in her article "Why young teens need real periods–not the Pill."

> "Making hormones is not easy. It requires regular ovulation, and that can take a few years to become established. That's why the early years of menstruation are exactly the wrong time to take hormonal birth control…These girls are at risk for many of the side effects of hormonal birth control including impaired bone density, altered brain structure, increased risk for depression, and suppressed libido. Side effects occur partly from the synthetic hormones themselves and partly from lack of girls' own estrogen and progesterone…When we shut down ovulation with hormonal birth control, we rob girls of the hormones they need for metabolism, bone health, cardiovascular health, mood, and more."

Another side effect of the widespread use of the contraceptive pill is that it has a detrimental impact on the balance of gut flora which is essential for a healthy digestive system.

The contraceptive pill has been in widespread use for more than 50 years, throughout the world, and is one of the major medications that is exported to third world countries as medical aid. You may be surprised at how much tax money and independent charitable donations are spent on contraceptive pills, condoms, formula, milk, and other such supplies. The female hormones that women consume on a daily basis are flushed from her system via her urine, and in cities with closed-loop water recycling systems, this means that it is flushed down the toilet and often taken away to water recycling systems, which clean and purify the water for use again. In a closed-loop system, water may recycle more than 40 times from tap to toilet to treatment plant and back again. Rather than removing the synthetic female hormones from the water that is deemed safe to drink, these hormones are actually concentrated and accumulate.

Anyone drinking this water, male or female, young or old, is being exposed to constant levels of female hormones, designed to mimic pregnancy and prevent ovulation. This has been linked to low sperm counts found in many males, and may also contribute to infertility issues in women, as sensitive women may be reacting to the chemicals in the contraceptive pill without even consciously taken them.

Where the water is not recycled, it is dumped into natural water sources such as rivers and seas, often contaminating underground aqueducts. When we consider that these hormones have been taken on a daily basis by millions of women worldwide for decades, then it is hardly surprising that ecologists have observed severe changes in fish and amphibious creatures such as frogs and crocodile (whose habitats are the contaminated water). The males are being born with deformed genitalia, or female reproductive systems, in some ecosystems very few males, have been observed, and many of them are incapable of reproduction.

Since the earth on which we live is a closed system, nothing that is thrown away ever really goes anywhere, and pollutants in our environment also affect human beings. Certain pesticides and chemicals leached from plastics have also been associated with mimicking female hormones, and some indigenous communities that live in environments with high levels of exposure to such chemicals have reported low birth rates of male children, sterility, and many genital-related deformities.

Many women who have been on the contraceptive pill for a significant amount of time find it difficult to achieve pregnancy immediately after quitting the pill. It often takes up to two years to detoxify the body of artificial chemicals and for hormone levels and periods to readjust, especially if the woman was never given the opportunity to experience and develop normal menstruation as an adolescent.

There are other methods of contraception, such as the contraceptive patches. They release the same hormones as the pill and work in the same way. There is also a uterine implant made of copper, which kills sperm. However, there have been reports of dangerous levels of copper toxicity associated with this method, in addition, any item inserted into the uterus, (including devices which vibrate, to prevent implantation of a fertilized egg), increase the risk of introducing bacteria or infection into the womb. Some of these devices have also been known to migrate, causing internal damage, discomfort, and on rare occasions permanent (rather than temporary) sterility in women.

Condoms are a popular choice. Countless tax dollars and charitable donations are spent on condoms every year which are distributed via free clinics and in third world aid shipments. They are the first means of contraception that most people turn to. However, condoms are more than just physical barriers. According to ancient Ayurvedic and Taoist philosophies, during the sexual act, there is a profound exchange of energy which can both enhance and deplete vitality in the individual depending upon the quality of the relationship between the parties involved. In its purest form, sexual intercourse was identified as connecting the participants with the creative life forces of the universe. This would result in the manifestation of new physical life in the form of the growing fetal body for a child's soul, but also produce a creative and life-giving energy which could be harnessed to rejuvenate and heal the body and manifest creative potential in other areas of their lives.

Every woman absorbing the sperm of her partner absorbs the energy of the male at climax, his emotional, karmic, physical and spiritual energy, affecting her own energy and manifesting in her body and her psyche. A man with poor health, such as an STD, shares that negative energy pattern with his partner, likewise, a violent or emotionally unattached man will also affect the psyche and self-image of the woman. Scientists have discovered male DNA in the bodies of many women (even those who have not had male children or aborted/miscarried pregnancies (mothers carry their children's DNA within their body for the rest of their lives), which they believe has entered the mother's body and been absorbed through past sexual relationships. This discovery could indicate that a woman is absorbing a part of every man that she has had intercourse. Some women who have experienced fertility issues explore deep womb cleansing techniques and therapies in an attempt to rid themselves of the physical and energetic residue of past sexual relationships which they feel may be negatively affecting their reproductive capacities.

Although it is unclear whether a condom which acts as a barrier to sperm could prevent the long-term receptivity of the woman to the energy and DNA of her sexual partners, it certainly seems to have affected her emotional attachment.

With the prevalence of condoms in mainstream society (as opposed to the limitation of their use to their original place in brothels by sex workers), coupled with other factors, such as mainstream media and so-called popular culture, there seems to have been a degradation in the intimacy of relationships which contain a sexual encounter.

More often, women are choosing to seek quantity over quality of sexual relationships in their lives. Rather than being a positive gain in women's rights to sexual freedom, this choice lacks the fulfilling and spiritually satisfying consequences of a union base upon mutual respect, love, and commitment.

Sex deserves to be sacred, and women owe it to themselves to retain the value of sexual intimacy, as do men. It is beyond time that society redressed its message to men that sex is anything other than profound. It saddens me that such a vulgar and empty value of sex has been offered to men as their only option, rather than enlightening them of the deep satisfaction of a sexual bond cemented by love and devotion, that is mutually beneficial to themselves, their partners and to the whole of society.

I do not mean to suggest that sex should be banished to past paradigms of shame or embarrassment, but rather that the perspective of sex be elevated to acknowledge its sacred (divine) nature. Sex should be holy, especially when it is the beginning of a new soul's incarnation on earth, and it should be spiritual, emotionally, physically, and psychologically rewarding to all involved. It should be an act of appreciation and gratitude, a celebration and honor of life and all its unique and marvelous gifts, above all, it should be a natural expression of love.

Natural Alternatives

Natural methods of contraception include herbal formulas which have been traditionally used in many cultures throughout history. Most of these do not have a track record of 100% prevention, however. Herbal contraceptives work in a variety of ways; some are used to prevent ovulation, others to create an inhospitable environment for implantation within the uterus and others are used to bring on a late period within two or so weeks of it having been missed.

Sterility Promoters as listed in Susan Weeds "Wise Woman Herbal for the Childbearing Years" include Stone seed root (Lithospermum ruderal), Jack-in-the-Pulpit root (Arisaema triphyllum), and thistles. Implantation Preventers include wild carrot seeds (Daucus carota), smart-weed leaves (Polygonum hydropiper). Menstrual Promoters include ginger (Zingiber) Tansy leaves (Tanacetum Vulgare), pennyroyal leaves (Hedeoma pulegioides), large doses of vitamin C, angelica root, cohosh, feverfew, hyssop, lovage root, rue, mugwort plant, mistletoe leaves, Peruvian bark, amongst others. Uterine Contractors include cotton root bark (Gossypium) and blue cohosh root (Caulophyllum thalictroides).

If you would like to consider using any herbal methods of contraception, then I suggest consulting a herbal medicine practitioner trained and specializing in the female reproductive matter, since all herbal medicines have a variety of medicinal compounds. It is essential to get expert advice on dosages, sourcing of high-quality uncontaminated organic plant material, and what plants are suitable for your body, allergies, ongoing medical conditions and to consider any other medication you may be taking as they can interact with one another.

Another very effective method of natural contraception is the use of diluted Neem oil as a lubricant as a vaginal pessary prior to sex, as Neem oil is a natural spermicide. In India, some men consume Neem leaves in order to lower or eradicate their sperm count. Neem is a natural anti-parasitic and is often taken internally to eradicate intestinal parasites. As an oil, it can be used as a treatment for vaginal yeast infections, fungal infections, and dandruff. It is, however, very bitter so be careful to wash your hands. Abstinence is, of course, the most effective form of contraception.

Fertility Awareness

Knowing when you ovulate can help to determine which days of the month you are likely to be fertile and could be at-risk of becoming pregnant. There are certain signals from a woman's body that she can learn to read, which let her know when she is ovulating. A woman's temperature is notably higher during ovulation and can be recorded via thermometer, and her vaginal discharge is thought to become more elastic...like egg whites. It may be worth noting down temperature and vaginal discharge consistency in your menstrual journal as you map your three menstrual cycles, as it may help to provide further insight on fertility and conception for the future.

A healthy woman ovulates one day per menstrual cycle, and the egg which is released can remain fertile for three days. However, sperm can survive inside of a woman's body for five days, which means that to avert the possibility of pregnancy, the rhythm method of natural contraception suggests avoiding sexual intercourse from a minimum of five days before expected ovulation. Some methods suggest abstaining from sex for a ten day period during this fertile time. It is worth investigating if this method is one that you are interested in implementing. However, it is not 100% effective and is often combined with barrier methods.

We are naturally programmed to ovulate with the full moon "The pineal gland in our brain sends messages to our ovary, by hormones, to release an egg based on the amount of light our brain senses in the night when we are asleep. At the point of most light in the night, the full moon, we …ovulate." The spiritual practice of menstruation by Jane Hardwicke Collings.

Pregnancies have been reported after sexual intercourse at various stages throughout the cycle, even sex during menstruation. "Each woman has the potential to ovulate a second time in her cycle when the phase of the moon is the same as it was when she was born - her lunar return. This is called the Lunar Ovulation" says "The spiritual practice of menstruation" by Jane Hardwicke Collings. Conversely, the likelihood of pregnancy for those seeking to conceive can be greatly increased by understanding the natural rhythms of the woman's fertility cycle and timing intercourse with ovulation.

Fertility awareness is an essential part of body literacy that most women would benefit from fluency in and should be taught to young girls as they transition from prepubescents into adolescents, to prepare them for their lives as healthy empowered and fully conscious womb-men.

Sanitary Products

There are an abundant variety of brands and products available to help women contain their monthly bleed so that they can continue with their daily lives and duties without disruption, however, in truth, the choices are somewhat limited. Disposable products come in two basic options, tampons or pads. Although it is possible now to find organic cotton products, the majority of "feminine hygiene products such as tampons and sanitary pads are an oft-ignored source of a variety of potentially toxic ingredients, including genetically modified organisms and pesticides" states Dr. Mercola in "4 Ways to Honor The Power Of Menses." And "each conventional sanitary pad contains ingredients found in about four plastic bags," says Andrea Donsky, founder of Naturally Savvy and co-author of "Label Lessons: Your Guide to a Healthy Shopping Cart." Many tampons are made of synthetic fibers that have been bleached to give them that "clean" look that appeals to most consumers. But the Environmental Protection Agency (EPA) has proven that using any products with chlorine increases the risk of cancer exponentially.

As well as the potentially carcinogenic chemicals, the use of tampons also increases the risk of exposure to toxic shock syndrome; there are also some people who believe that the use of tampons prevents the release of all of the menstrual blood.

Retained menstrual blood can be the cause of much discomfort and even infection; vaginal steams are often recommended to assist in cleansing the womb. Another alternative is a moon cup, a small chalice shaped device that is inserted into the vagina to collect menstrual blood. While these are also made of plastic, they are reusable, however, not every woman finds them comfortable, and it is important to make sure that they are inserted correctly to avoid distortion. Moon cups are available in a variety of shapes and sizes, and it may be necessary to shop around to find out what works best for you.

According to Dr. Joseph Mercola, "the average American woman uses up to 16,800 tampons in her lifetime—or as many as 24,360 if she's on estrogen replacement therapy". The use of disposable sanitary products in such vast quantities has had a devastating effect on the environment. Most tampons and even some sanitary pads get flushed down the toilet and washed out to sea. According to Marine Debris Specialist Nicholas Mallos, in 2012, during the Ocean Conservancy's International Coastal Clean-up, nearly 40,000 tampons and applicators were found internationally along beaches and waterways worldwide

An alternative to disposable sanitary towels are reusable menstrual pads made from cotton, which can be soaked, washed and reused. These can be bought online and in some health food shops. There are also many free patterns on the internet; so that you can make your own, share with friends and family, or even start your own business. Menstrual pads can be made from recycled materials such as old cotton, flannel shirts, and sweatshirts, and waterproof liners can be added to prevent spillage and can be used to make bags to carry the used pads when out in public, very similar to those used for fitted reusable cotton nappies for babies and young infants.

Menstrual Medicine and Blood Magic

Blood has always been associated with vital energy, life, power, and magic. Blood sacrifices have been offered in ceremonies for centuries, from the sacrifices of lives in ancient cultures to the self-sacrifice of the warriors of Native America in the well-known annual Sun Dance. Self-mutilation has been viewed as an initiation into a culture, and as part of coming of age rituals for men and women in various cultures, from ritual scarring, piercing and tattooing to circumcision and cock-holding. However, the first blood, the blood of life, and continued life have always been moon blood, womb blood. The blood of womb-men.

Menstrual blood is the only blood that flows without trauma, it is a natural and healthy cleansing blood, a marking of cycles, a marking of fertility, and a gift, for it is blood given freely, without pain or suffering or sacrifice of life. Menstrual blood is the blood of life. Not death. It is the only blood which flows without a wound. Menstrual blood is sacred and has always been regarded as such.

The first blood offerings were the gifts that women gave of themselves, returning their blood, and the life force that their blood imbued, to the earth and the Great Mother that they worshiped, appreciated and depended upon. "Three or four thousand years ago the gods began a migration from the lakes, forests, rivers, and mountains into the sky, becoming the imperial overlords of nature rather than its essence of nature." "Sacred Economics: Money, Gift, and Society in the Age of Transition" by Charles Eisenstein.

Menstrual blood was once considered, unsurprisingly, even logically, to be the basis of life. The Maoris stated explicitly, 'that human souls were made of menstrual blood, which when retained in the womb assumed human form and grew into a man.'

Africans said menstrual blood is 'congealed to fashion a man.'

In Hindu theory as the Great Mother creates, her substance becomes thickened and forms a curd or clot. This was the way she gave birth to the cosmos, and women employ the same method on a smaller scale.

Indians of South America said all mankind was made of 'moon blood' in the beginning.

In ancient Mesopotamia, they believed the Great Goddess Ninhursag made mankind out of clay and infused it with her "blood of life." THE SACRED POWER OF MENSTRUAL BLOOD by Goddess of Sacred Sex

The idea that the first man or woman was formed from clay, mixed with blood, (menstrual blood), and thus infused with the life-giving powers and properties of blood, has echoed throughout the origins of many cultures and societies.

From this belief, a lot of magical practices and techniques have originated. Amongst native African cultures, fetishes (models and figures) were created with clay and menstrual blood (later other forms of blood) to provide homes for spirits and entities charged with specific purposes such as protection, attracting wealth, promoting harmony and even providing fertility. Statues and figurines have been uncovered by archaeologists throughout Europe, Asia, Africa and the Middle East which are believed to be fertility charms, carved from bone and stone, stained with blood, and formed from clay mixed with blood, which were then hardened in ancient kilns. These charms may have been passed amongst communities for generations believed to be endowed with the magical ability to bless women with fertility, satisfying the hopes and longings for future children and families.

Many women exploring ancient traditions and embracing shamanic practices are experimenting with creating their own fertility charms, using their menstrual blood to empower the talismans and to link them personally to the individual's bodies and goals.

Menstrual blood has also been used for a variety of other purposes throughout the ages. Menstruation was intimately linked to sex; in the African-American-based folk spirituality of Hoodoo, and in the rituals of Italian and Sicilian witchcraft, a woman's menstrual blood was collected and added to the food of a man that she wished to attract to bind him to her in love and/or marriage.

Menstrual blood could also be substituted (it may originally have been the other way around) for any blood required in ritual, from ink to write sigils and charms to personalize spells or sign oaths and was used to fertilize the earth in ancient agricultural societies that depended upon fertile fields and abundant harvests.

Menstrual blood is life-giving and life-sustaining. It is an incredible nutrient to give to plants in the garden. Many women collect the soaking water from their menstrual pads or the blood collected in their moon cups to water their gardens and feed their house plants.

Some sources claim that menstrual blood was initially used as a drink for communion amongst witch covens. It is even suggested that it inspired Christian communion, in which wine was substituted to represent sacred blood, (the blood of Christ).

Many rituals in ancient Egypt involved the ingestion of menstrual blood mixed with wine, Egyptian Pharaohs became divine by ingesting 'the blood of Isis,' and the Celtic kings became gods by drinking the "red mead" of the Fairy Queen Mab. Norse mythology records that Thor reached the magic land of enlightenment and eternal life by bathing in a river filled with the menstrual blood of a 'giantesses.'

Within the ancient Taoist sexual mysteries, a woman's menstrual blood was considered to be extremely powerful. Taoists said a man could become immortal by absorbing menstrual blood, called red yin juice, from a woman's Mysterious Gateway. Chinese sages called this red juice the essence of Mother Earth, the yin principle that gives life to all things. It was claimed that the Yellow Emperor became a god by absorbing the yin juice of 1,200 women.

Within the ancient Hindu tantric traditions, special initiations of men are said to be given by knowledgeable women during their menstruation, who were able to initiate the men through the blood mysteries of the womb.

Within Kundalini traditions, a woman's cycle of fertility is seen to absorb a great deal of creative energy which is lost with each menstruation. When a woman reaches menopause, the creative energy is said to be absorbed by and accumulates inside of the women making her more powerful and wiser as she becomes a respected elder within the community.

The red dot (bhindi) worn by Hindu women between their eyes may originally have been painted with menstrual blood anointing the third eye chakra, according to The Spiritual Practice of Menstruation by Jane Hardwicke Collings http://www.moonsong.com.au/about.html

As well as "magical" use, menstrual blood has long been associated with healing and medicine. Recipes found written in hieroglyphics from ancient Egypt recommend applying menstrual blood to a woman's skin to promote beauty and remove the signs of aging, as a cure for sagging breast and even stretch marks.

Aboriginal women of Australia also knew of the incredible healing qualities of menstrual blood, long before modern medicine. Indigenous women would save their blood, and all the blood of the women of a community in one sacred place; this blood when dried was used on wounds and injuries to promote healing.

Menstrual blood was also mentioned in Traditional Chinese Medicine, and the medieval European nun Hildegard von Bingen who published medical texts believed the application of menstrual blood could cure leprosy.

Stem Cells

Modern science has recently made the discovery that menstrual blood contains stem cells, the mother cells from which all cells of the human body can be generated. Investigations into the application of stem cell technology are still relatively new, and the majority of research has been based on stem cells retrieved from aborted fetuses, or live bone marrow donations. However, the discovery of stem cells in menstrual blood, a trauma-less, victimless, and unlimited potential resource that each woman is gifted with every month provides an abundance of material. Menstrual blood can be genetically matched to a woman and her matrilineal line, (her genetic children and siblings), thus overcoming issues of rejection and incompatibility.

Researchers claim that using the unlimited potential of stem cells to generate healthy new tissue, will revolutionize the future of medicine and the treatment of conditions such as Parkinson's disease, Alzheimer's, cancer, and hundreds of other debilitating and life-threatening conditions. Some stem cell banks will offer to store the stem cells from menstrual blood for a fee, and it is not so different from cord blood banking, except that menstrual blood is produced every 28 days.

It seems that our ancestors may have had the wisdom of blood and its capacity for healing long before we even considered the possibility, however, misguided taboos may have suppressed the knowledge and application of this resource within Occidental culture until now.

Some modern women hoping to reclaim their ancient wisdom have been experimenting with ingesting their own menstrual blood and applying it to their skin in facials.

Women who are pregnant or experiencing lactational amenorrhea, (due to breastfeeding) may find that the first menstrual cycle they experience after the temporary absence to be more intense emotionally, as their body adjusts once again to hormonal fluctuations.

Conclusion

It is important to recognize the value and worth of our monthly menstrual cycles and to honor the sacred mystery that connects us to one another and our universe. By reclaiming menstruation from the stigma and taboos long associated with it and recognizing it for its potential life-affirming and healing capacity, we can feel honored once again to take up the mantle of womanhood when our menarche commences, rather suffering through ignorance and mislabeling menstruation a burden as opposed to a gift.

I encourage every woman to align herself with the natural rhythms of her environment and dedicate herself to the study of her own body's mysteries. Know thyself and know thy sisters, help others to embrace their femininity and their very powerful natures as women, and help us to provide positive body images and body wisdom to future generations, as our daughters mature into women and as we become wise crones.

Blessings

Bibliography

1. Red moon, Miranda Gray

2. Wise woman herbal for the childbearing years by Susan weed.

3. Sacred economics: money, gift, and society in the age of transition by Charles Eisenstein.

4. The Tao of fertility by Ni, Daoshing, Herko, Dana

5. The spiritual practice of menstruation by Jane Hardwicke Collings http://www.moonsong.com.au/about.html

6. "(Hildegard leprosy) history period – a look at menstruation through the ages in 15 fascinating facts" Yvette caster for metro.co.u

7. "Why young teens need real periods–not the pill," guest post by Dr. Lara Briden, Md

8. "The sacred power of menstrual blood" posted by goddess of sacred sex in the goddess blog (this post adapted from information provided by seven Swann Esha Bertrand from the fountain of life http://www.thefountainoflife.org/ adapted from 'women's encyclopedia of myths and secret' by Barbara Walker).

9. "4 ways to honor the power of menses" published on the Honeycolony website by Laura Anne Rowell

10. "The pill kills," a report based on research by Dr. Angela Lanfranchi and Dr. Phillip Ney

11. "The crone: women of age, wisdom, and power" by Barbara g. Walker

Did you enjoy this book?

Would you like to read more from Jemmais Keval-Baxter

The Ho'oponopono Doula™?

Visit: www.hooponoponodoula.com and sign up for the mailing list to receive a Free E-books and find out more information about workshops, books, and events.

Other books in the series include:

A Doula's Guide to Education

A Doula's Guide to Nutrition

A Doula's Guide to The Placenta

A Doula's Guide to Breastfeeding

Also by Jemmais Keval-Baxter

Ho'oponopono Birth: Ho'oponopono for Pregnancy and Childbirth (coming soon)

If you liked this book, please leave a review so that others can find it too.

About the Author

Mrs. Jemmais Keval-Baxter resides in Chile with her family. She is a Natural Childbirth Coach, Doula, Doula Trainer, Writer, and EFT Coach. For more information about her books and workshops, please consult her website at **www.hooponoponodoula.com.**

www.ingramcontent.com/pod-product-compliance
Lightning Source LLC
Chambersburg PA
CBHW060700280326
41933CB00012B/2255